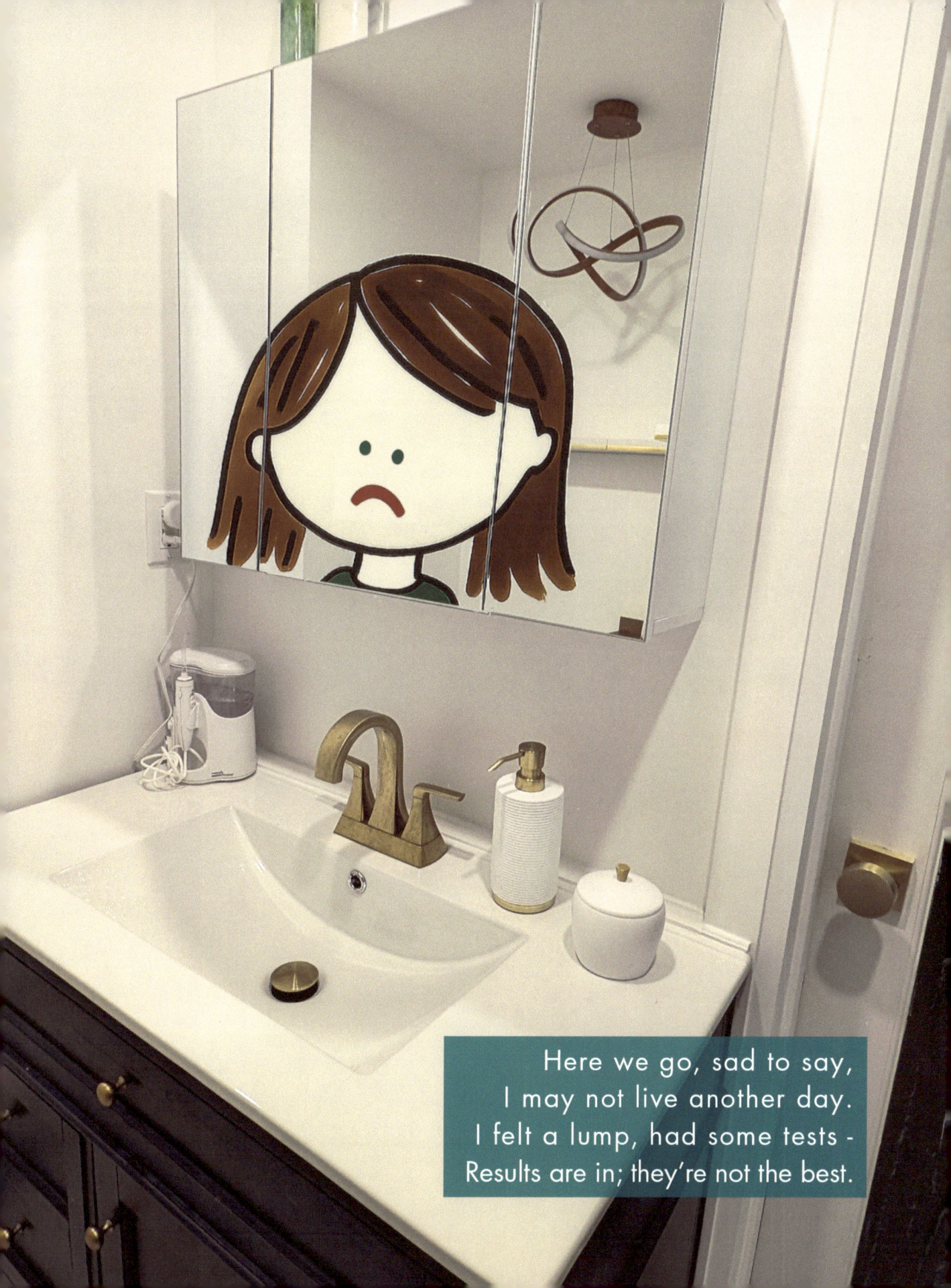

Here we go, sad to say,
I may not live another day.
I felt a lump, had some tests -
Results are in; they're not the best.

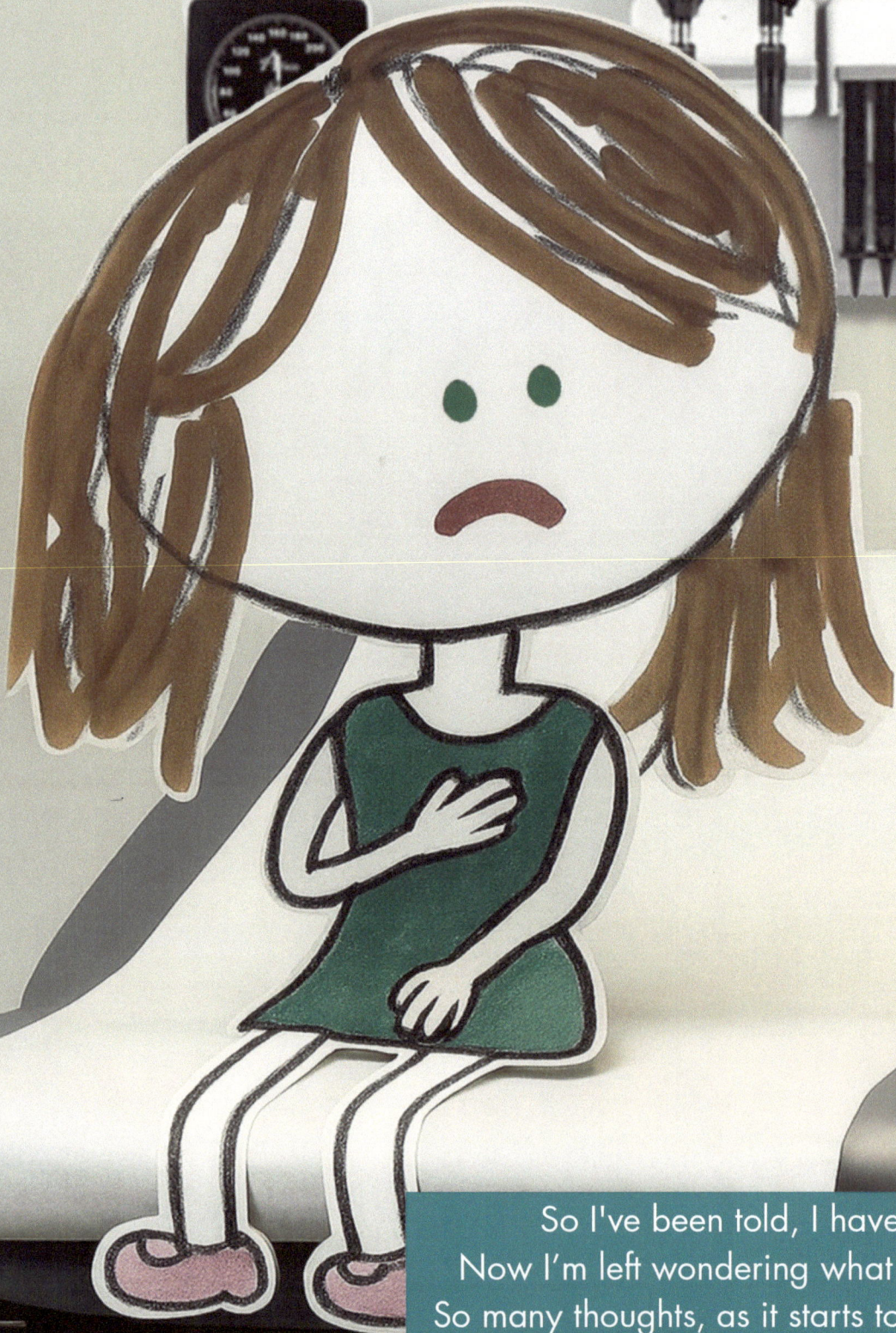

So I've been told, I have the "C."
Now I'm left wondering what will be?
So many thoughts, as it starts to invade -
Where do I start? I'm so afraid!

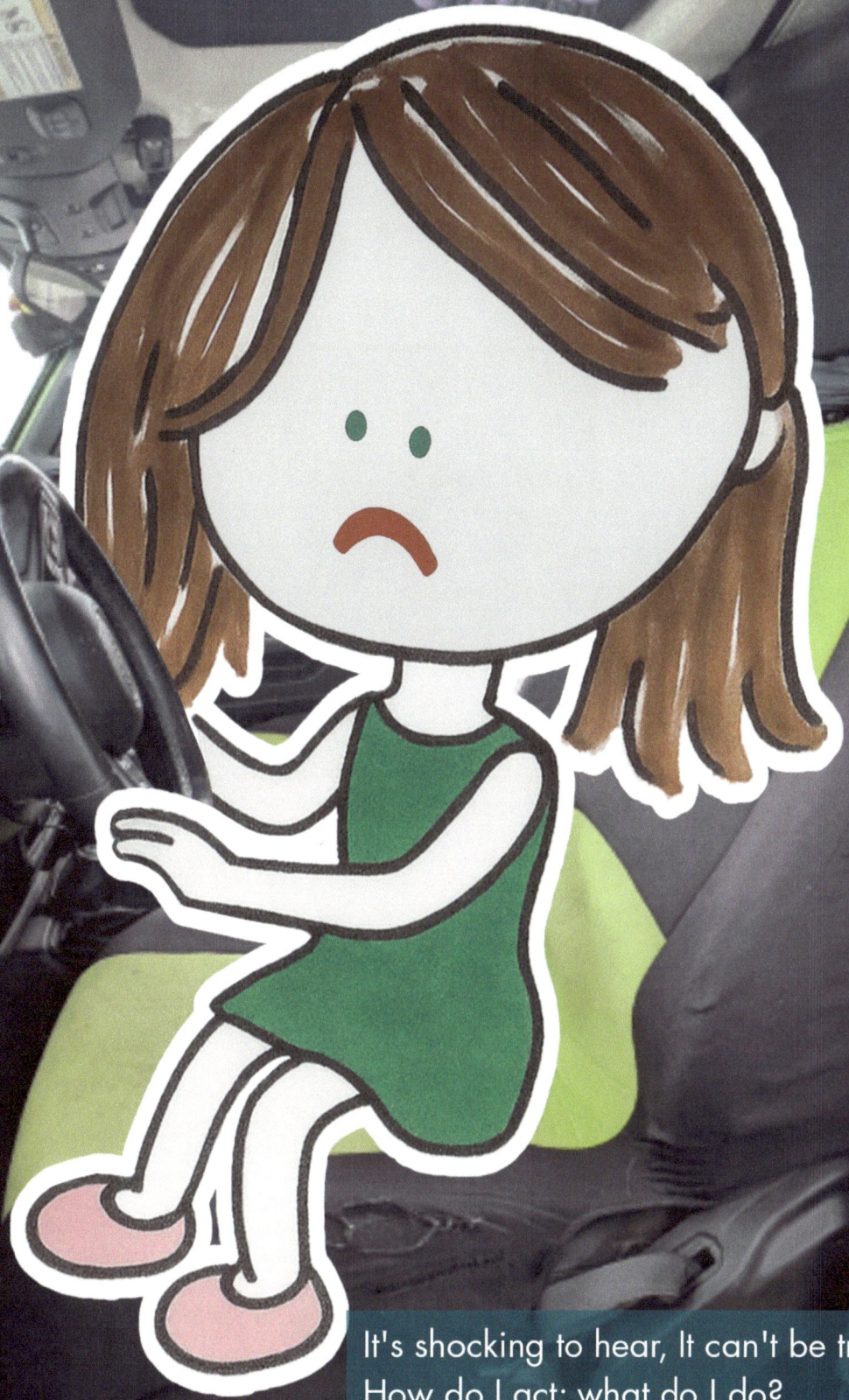

It's shocking to hear, It can't be true.
How do I act; what do I do?

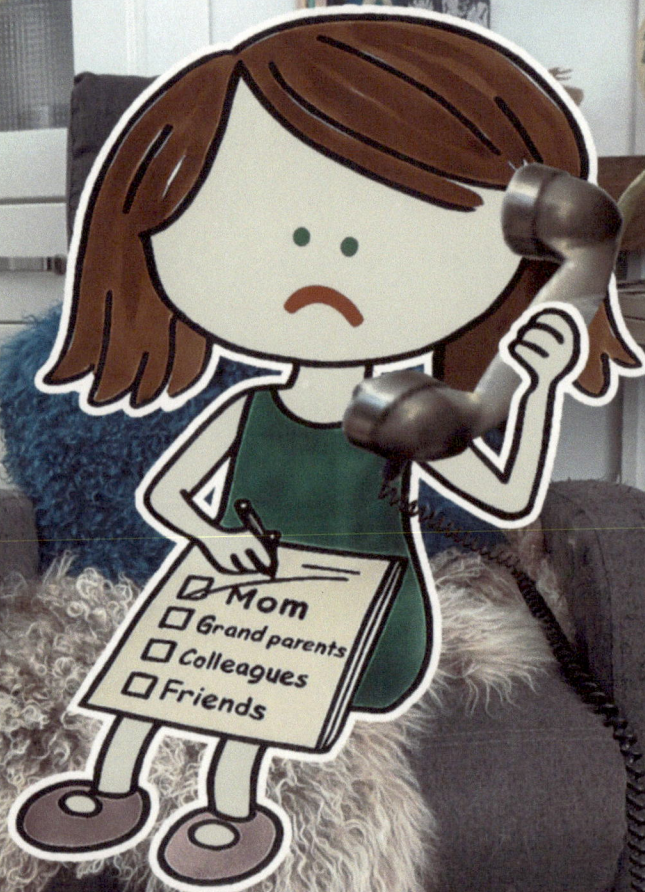

How do I tell my family and friends?
My life's now filled with twists, turns and bends.

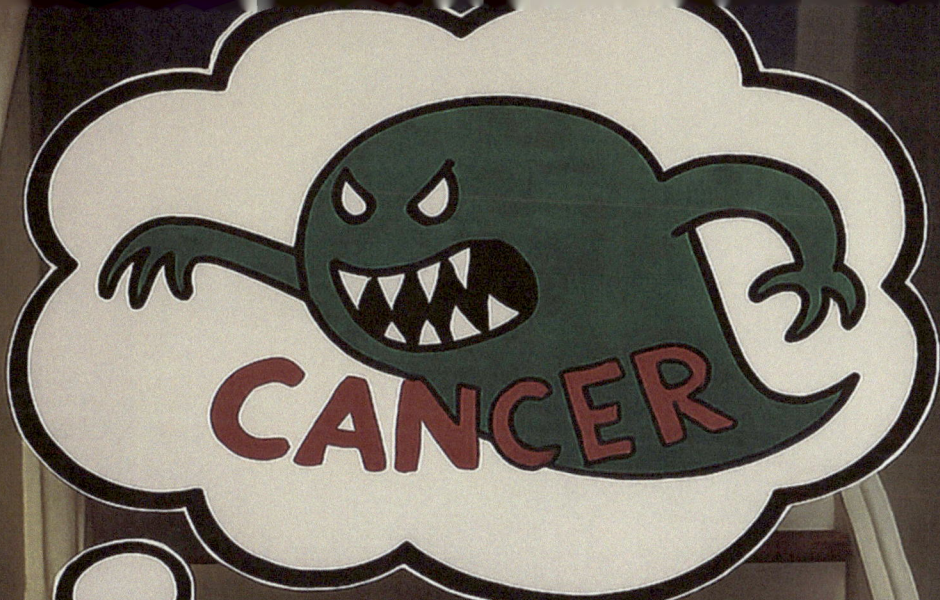

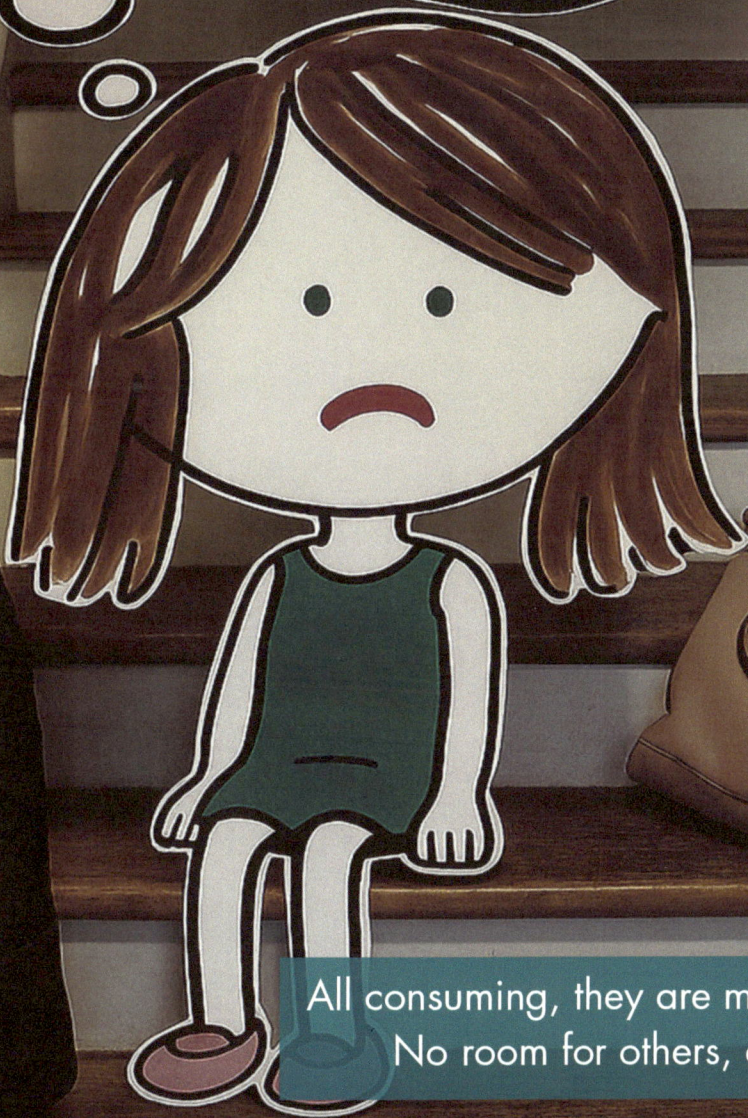

All consuming, they are my only thoughts -
No room for others, as my body rots.

MON	TUES	WED	THU	FRI
DOC	CHEM	TEST	TEST	XRAY
DOC	RN	CHEM	BLD	RAD
SURG	BLD	TEST	CHEM	RAD
RN	DOC	CHEM	RAD	

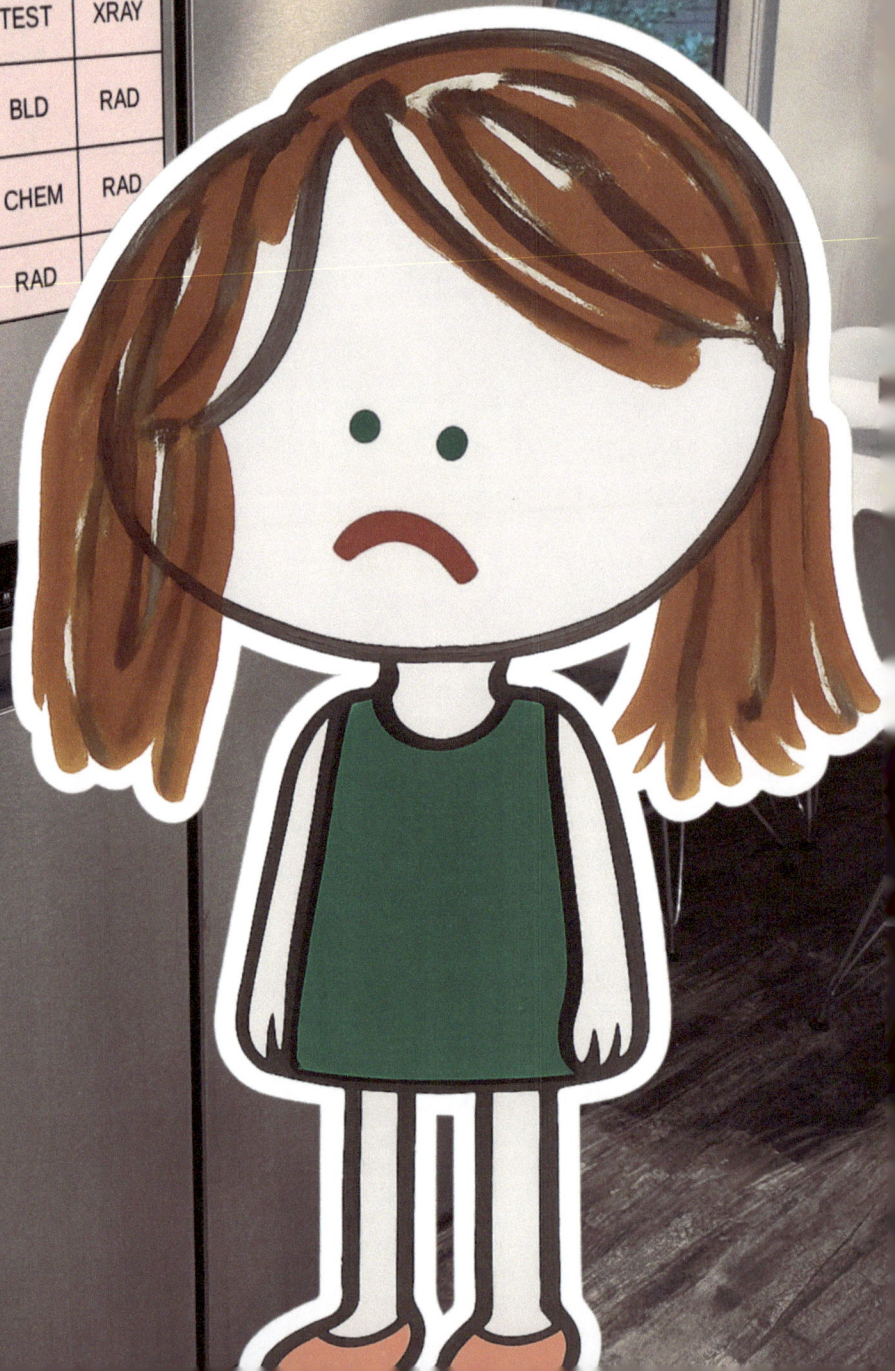

My days are filled with appointments galore
As I brace myself to start this war.
No time for work; no time for play -
These fucking visits take up my whole day!

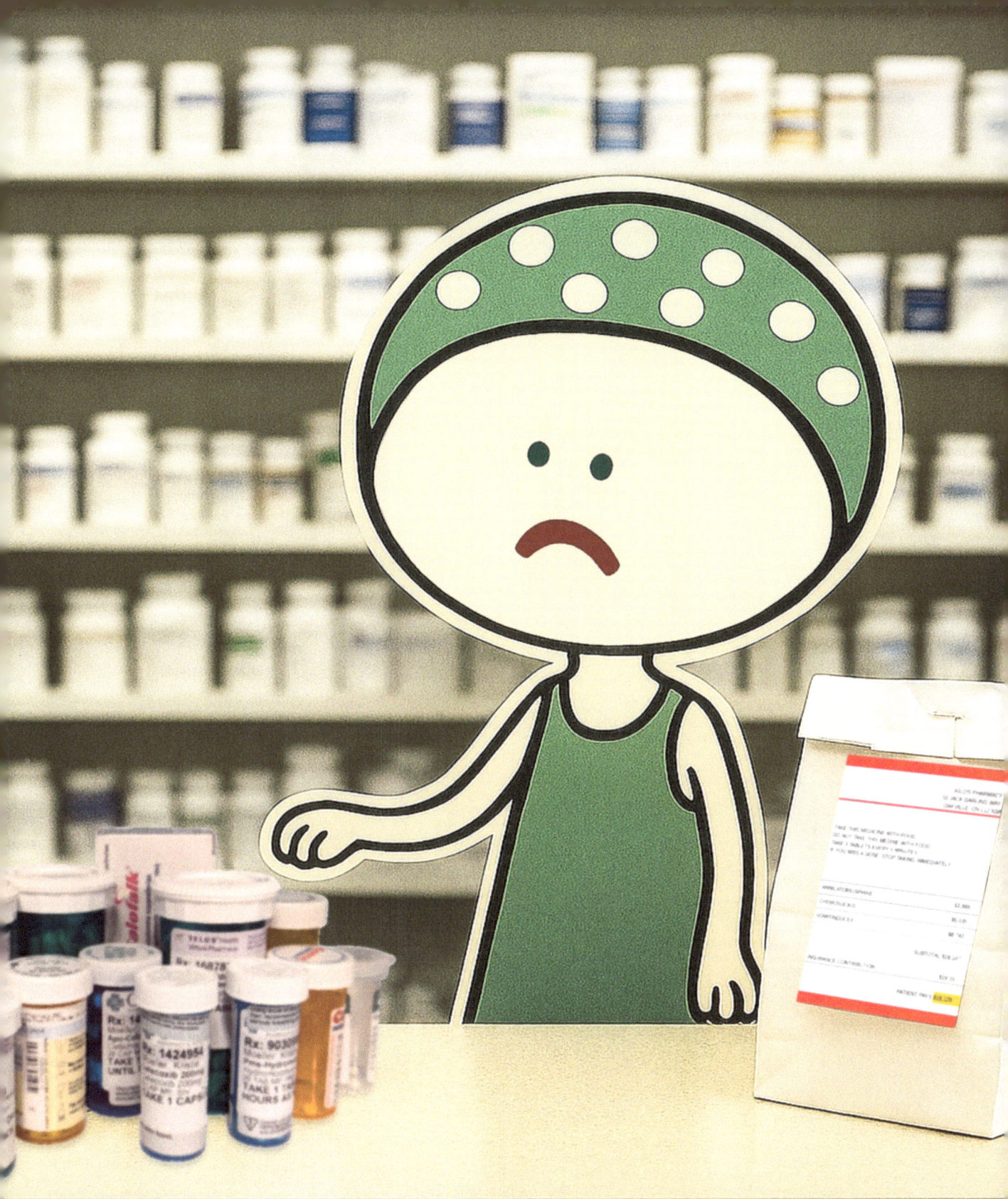

My Doctors prescribed such vicious drugs
Designed to annihilate all kinds of bugs.

The poison has taken my hair, taste and smell
And scrambled my brain as I tumble through hell.

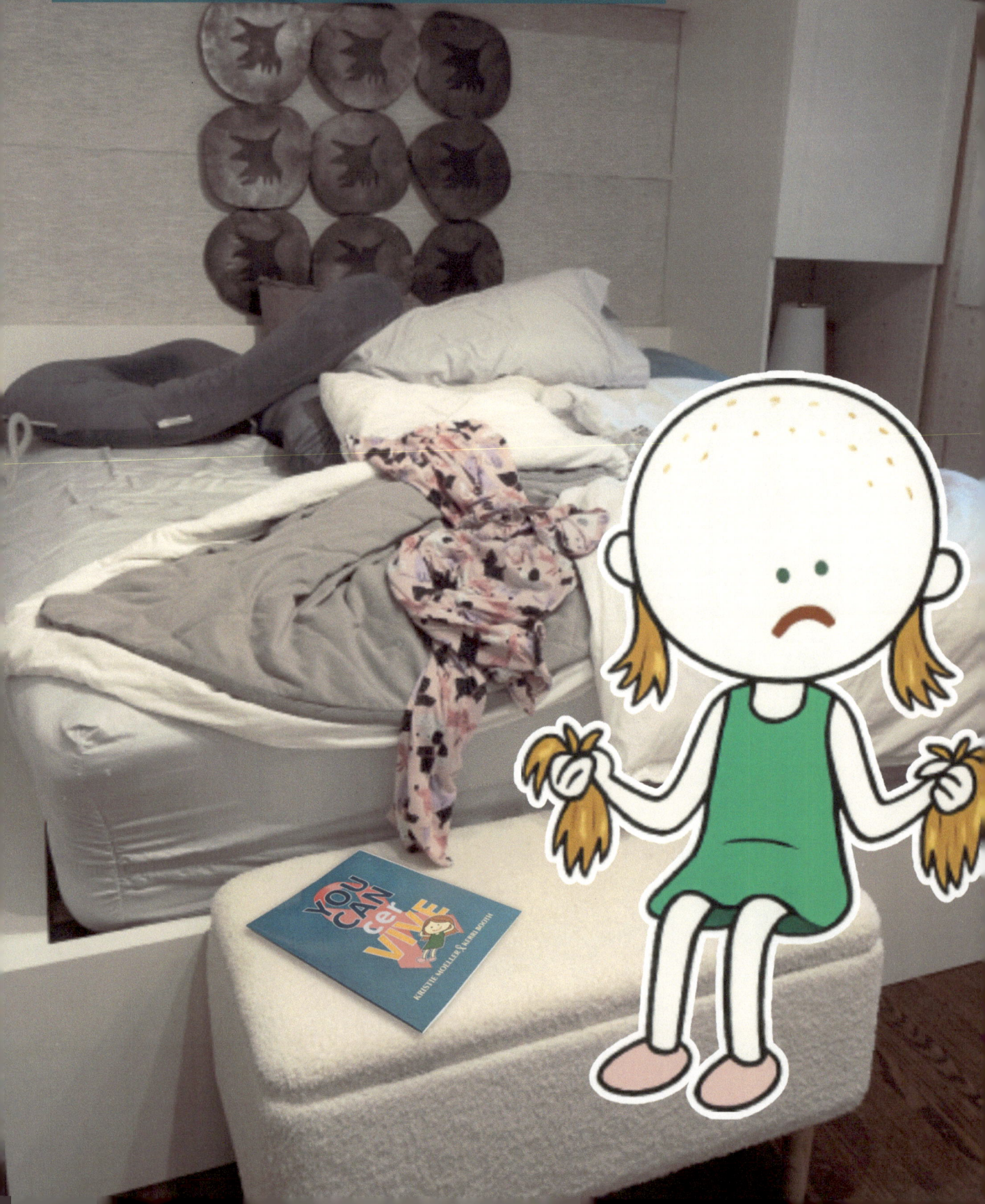

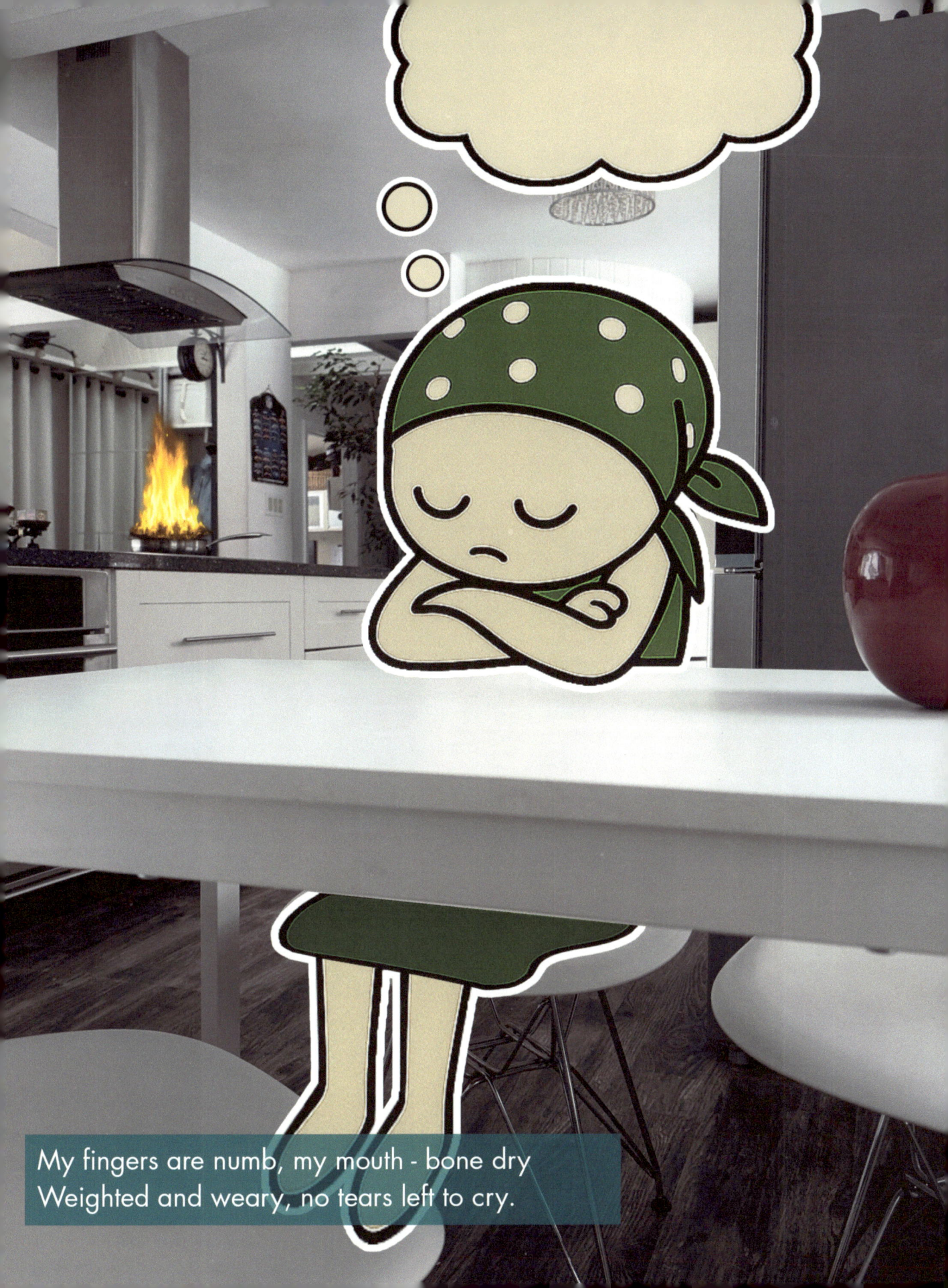

My fingers are numb, my mouth - bone dry
Weighted and weary, no tears left to cry.

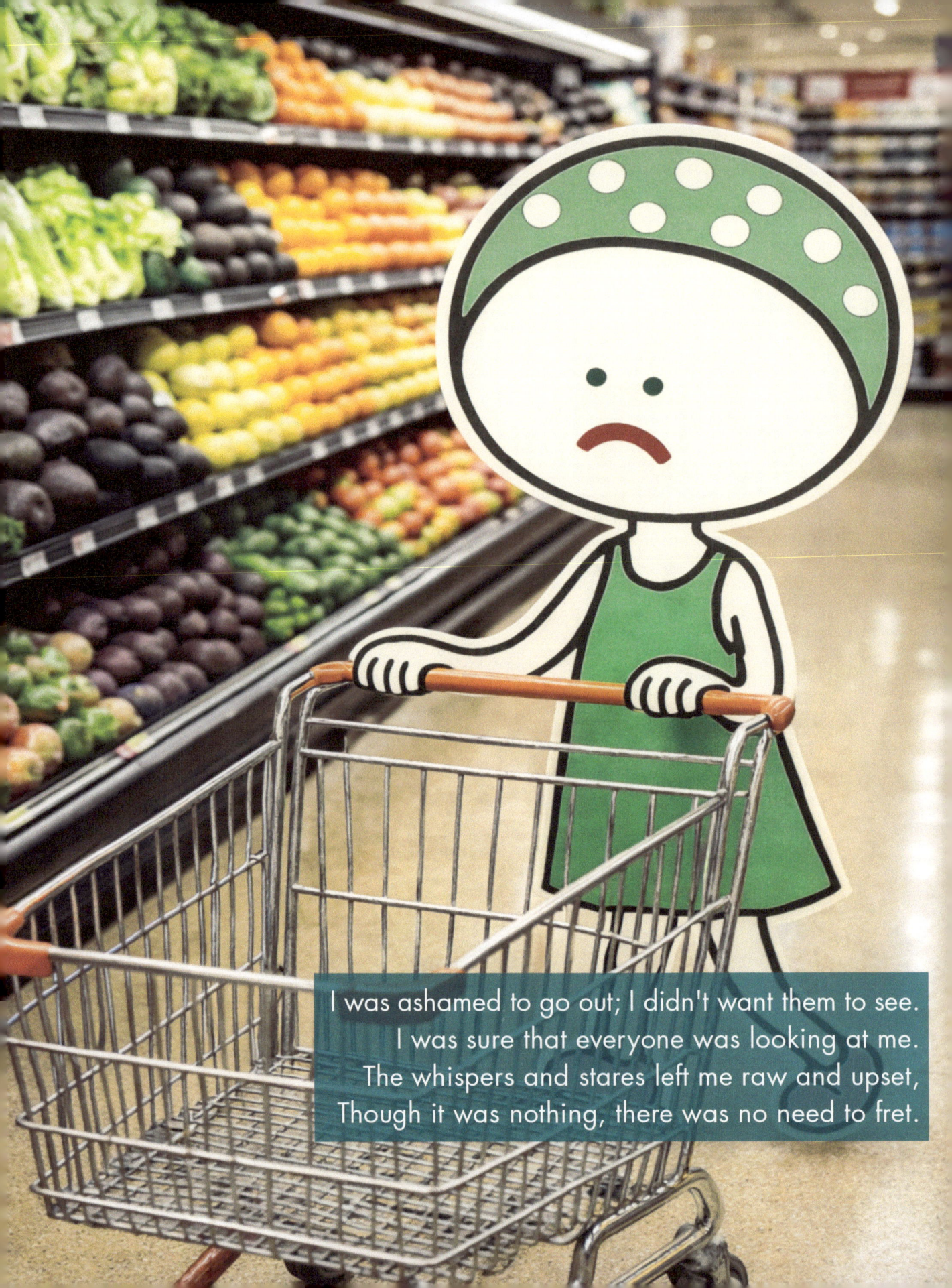

I was ashamed to go out; I didn't want them to see.
I was sure that everyone was looking at me.
The whispers and stares left me raw and upset,
Though it was nothing, there was no need to fret.

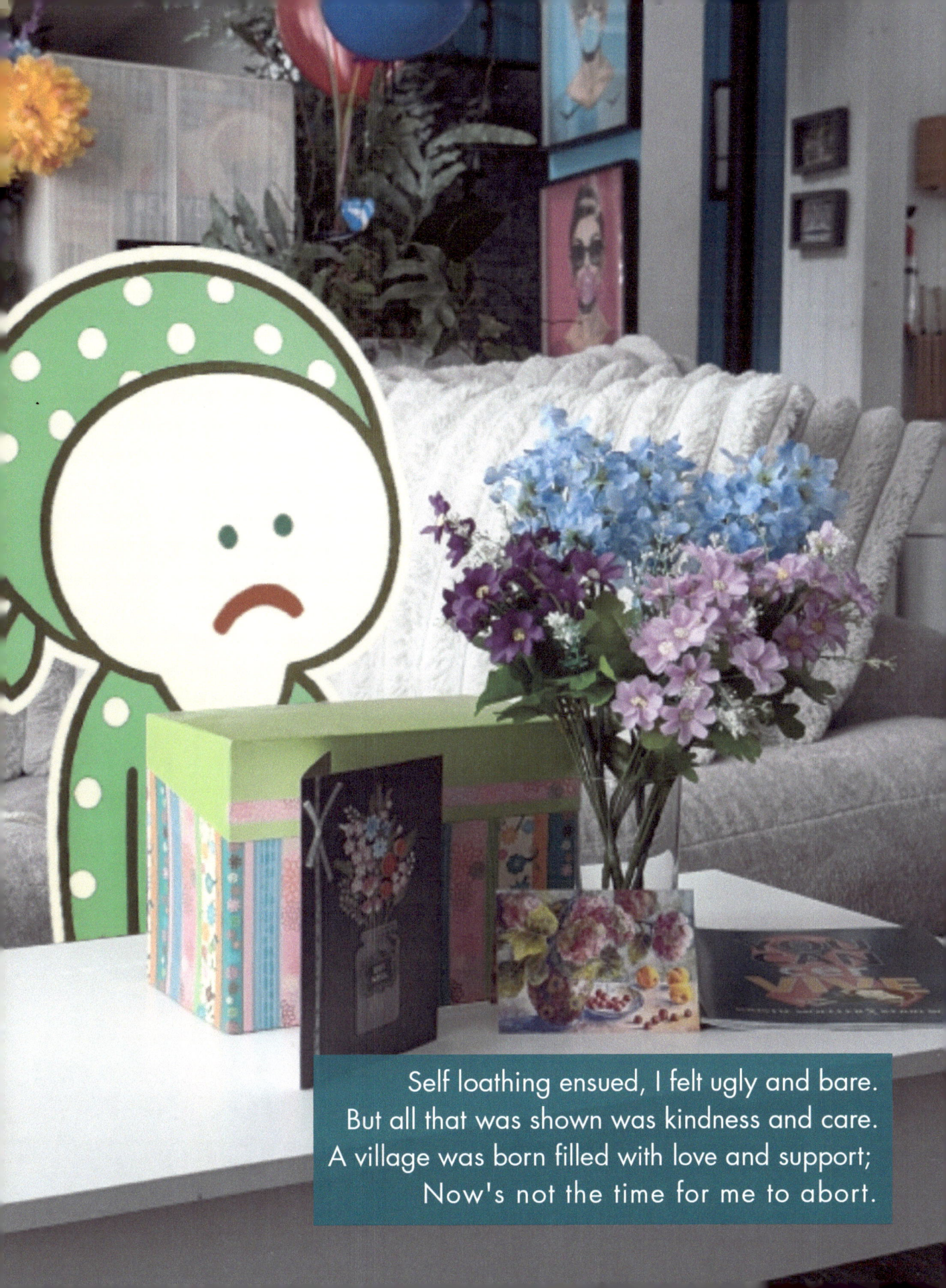

Self loathing ensued, I felt ugly and bare.
But all that was shown was kindness and care.
A village was born filled with love and support;
Now's not the time for me to abort.

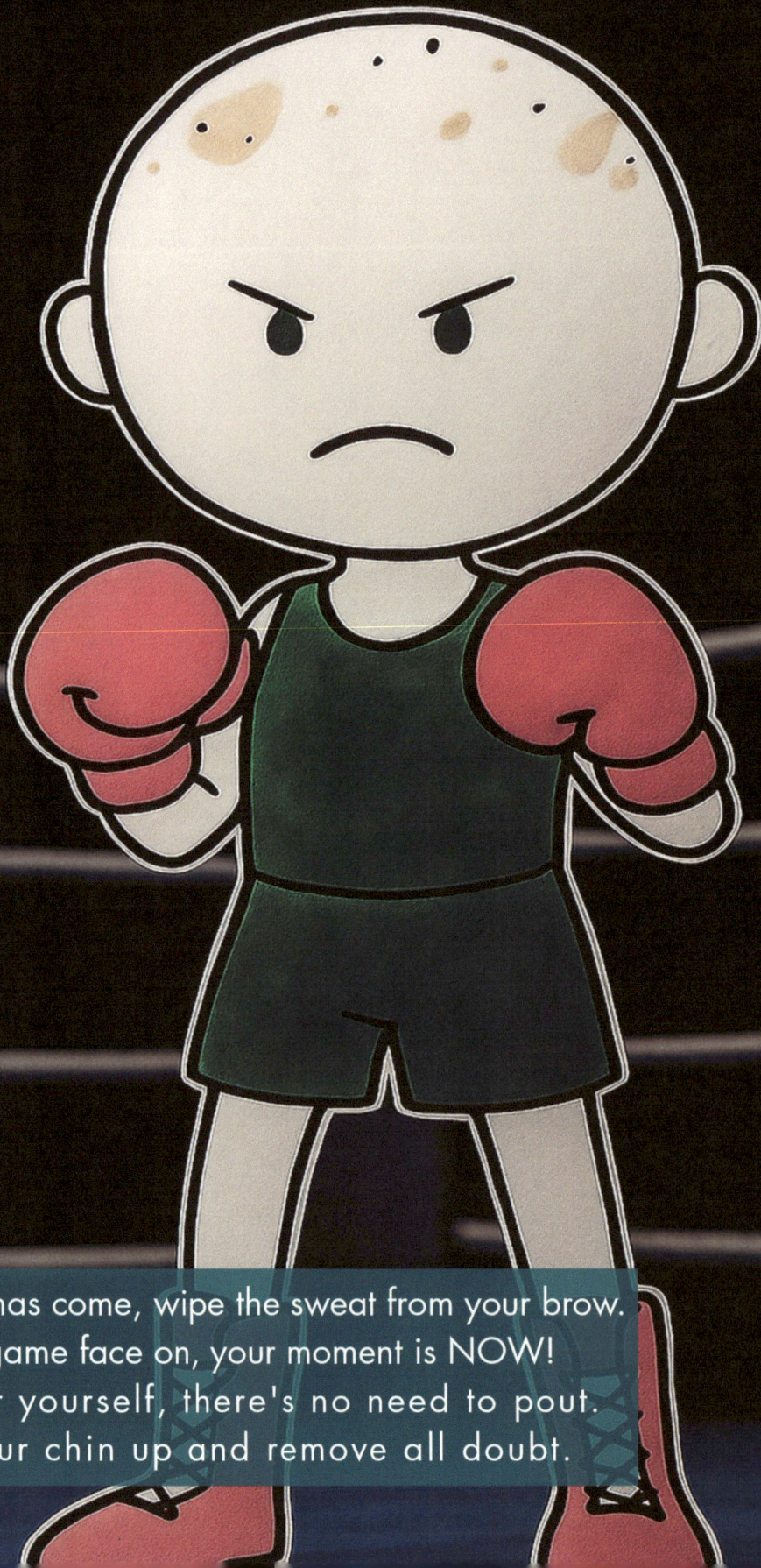

The time has come, wipe the sweat from your brow.
Put your game face on, your moment is NOW!
Get over yourself, there's no need to pout.
Keep your chin up and remove all doubt.

It's okay to be sad, angry and crass.
I know you'll kick this cocksucker's ass!
Take that negativity - toss it away.
It isn't welcome in your day to day.

MON	TUES	WED	THU	FRI
DOC	CHEM	TEST	TEST	XRAY
DOC	RN	CHEM	BLD	RAD
SURG	BLD	TEST	CHEM	RAD
RN	DOC	CHEM	RAD	BLD

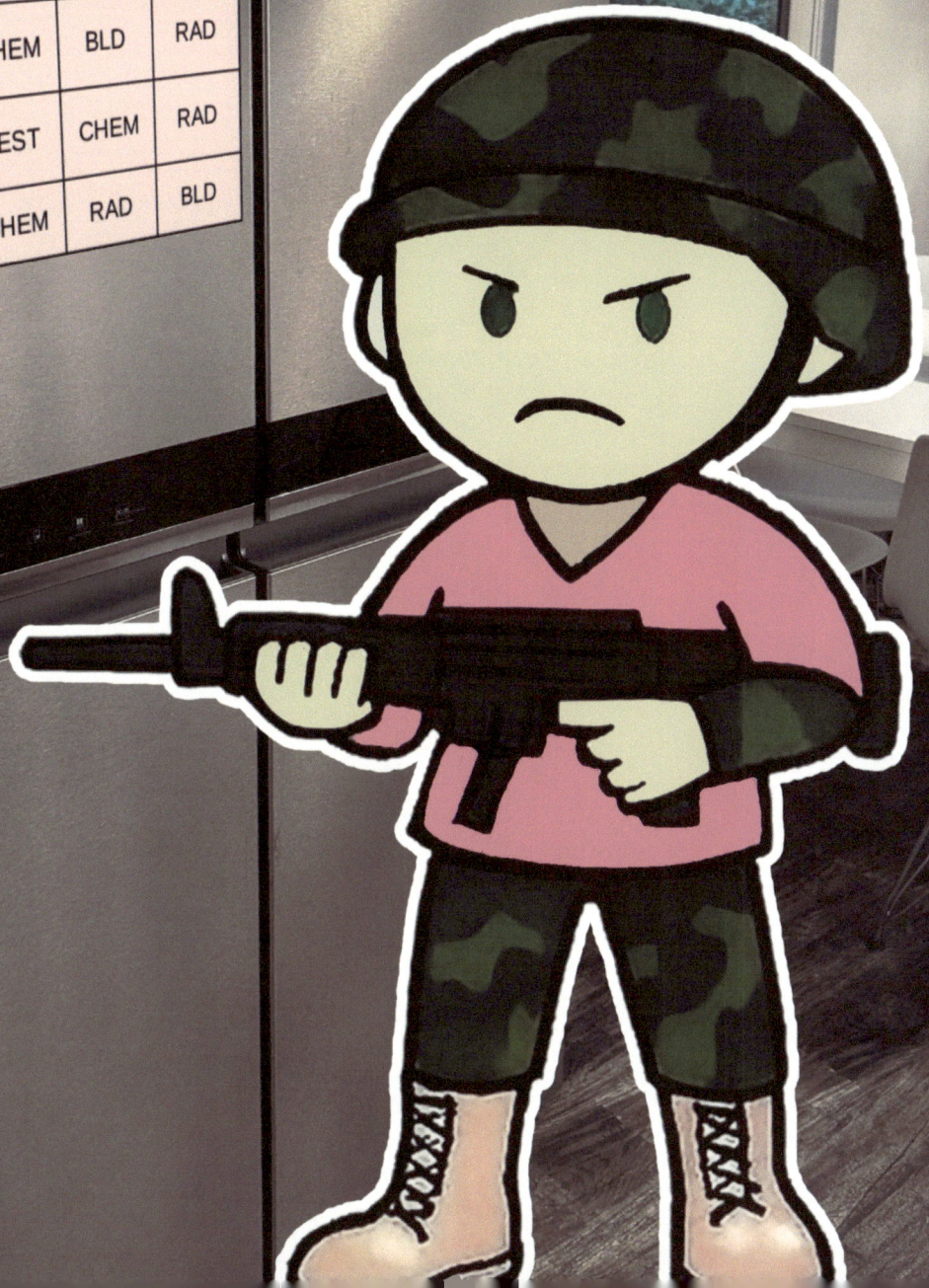

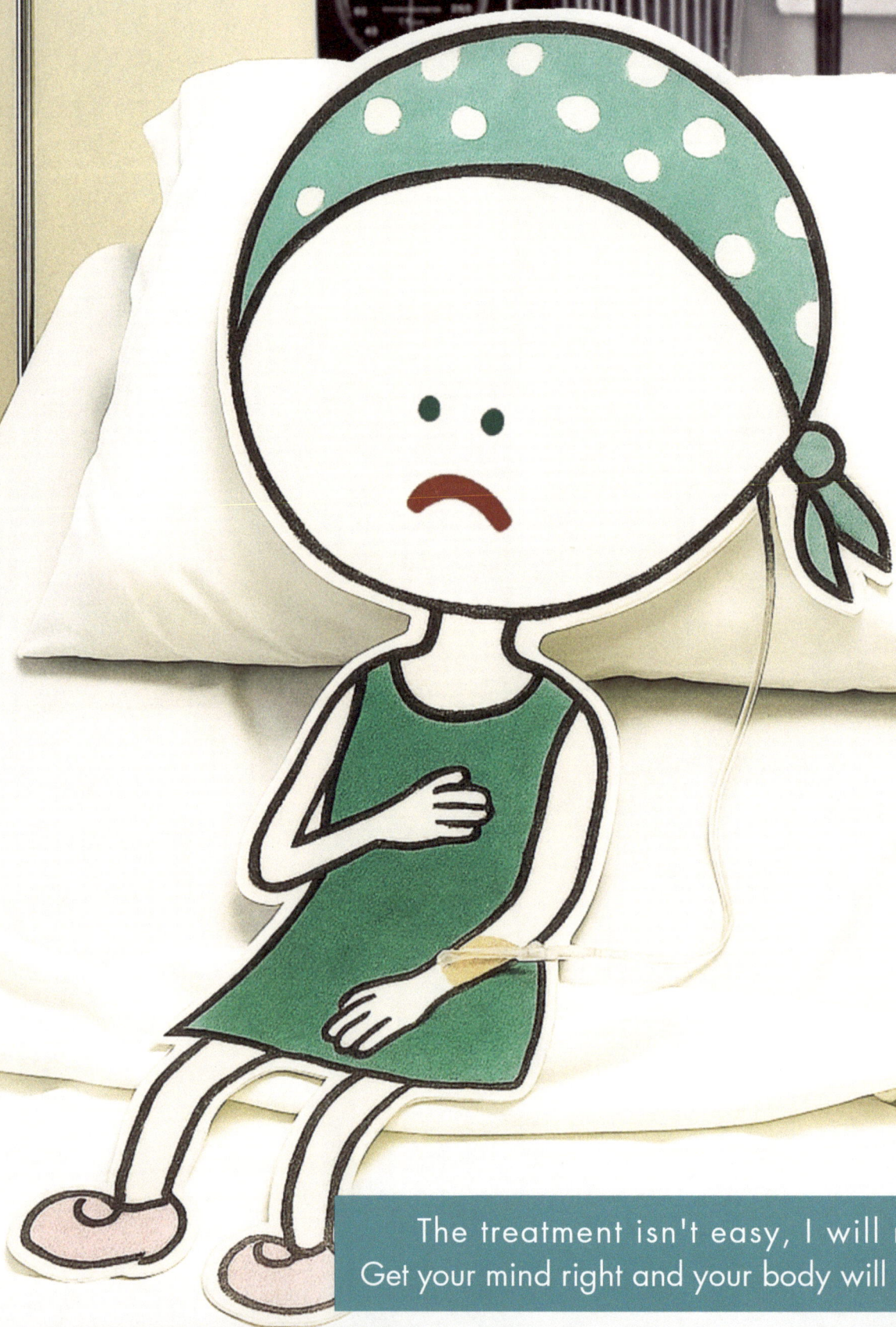

The treatment isn't easy, I will not lie.
Get your mind right and your body will comply.

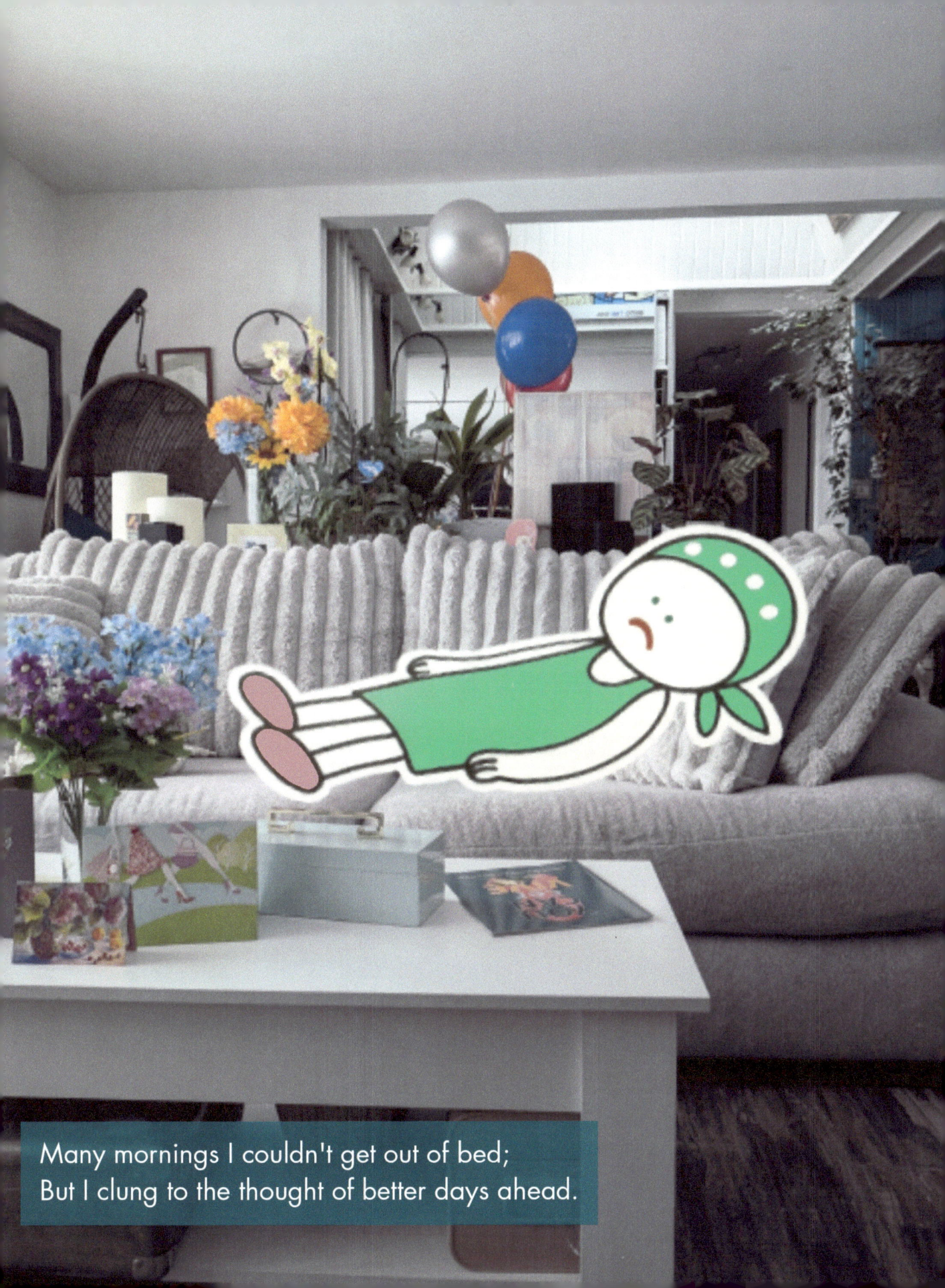

Many mornings I couldn't get out of bed;
But I clung to the thought of better days ahead.

Much better than my first time around.
Side effects, more bearable - or so I've found.
And when you find yourself on the brink;
Please remember, you're stronger than you think!

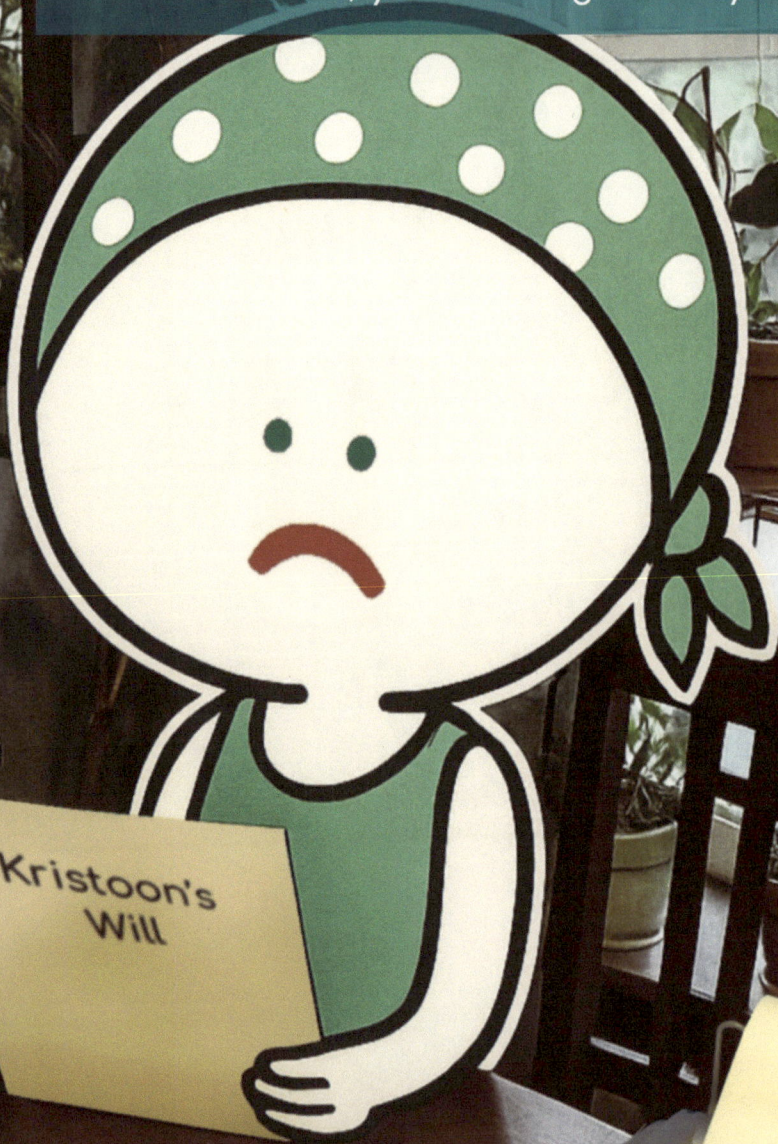

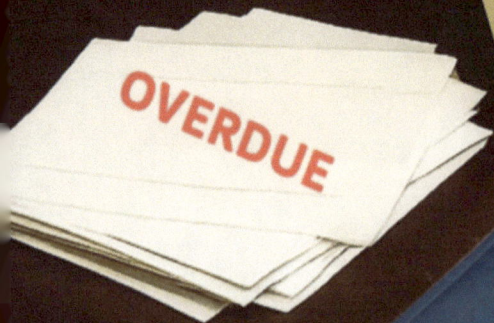

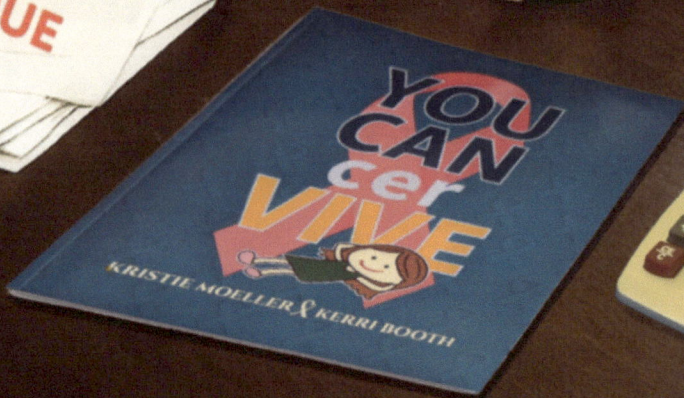

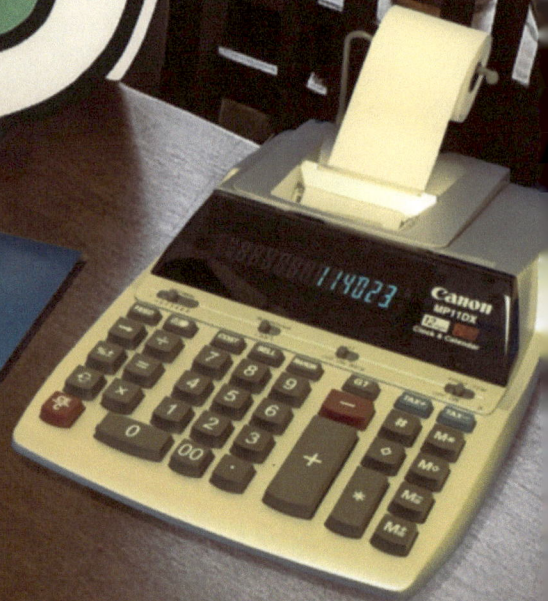

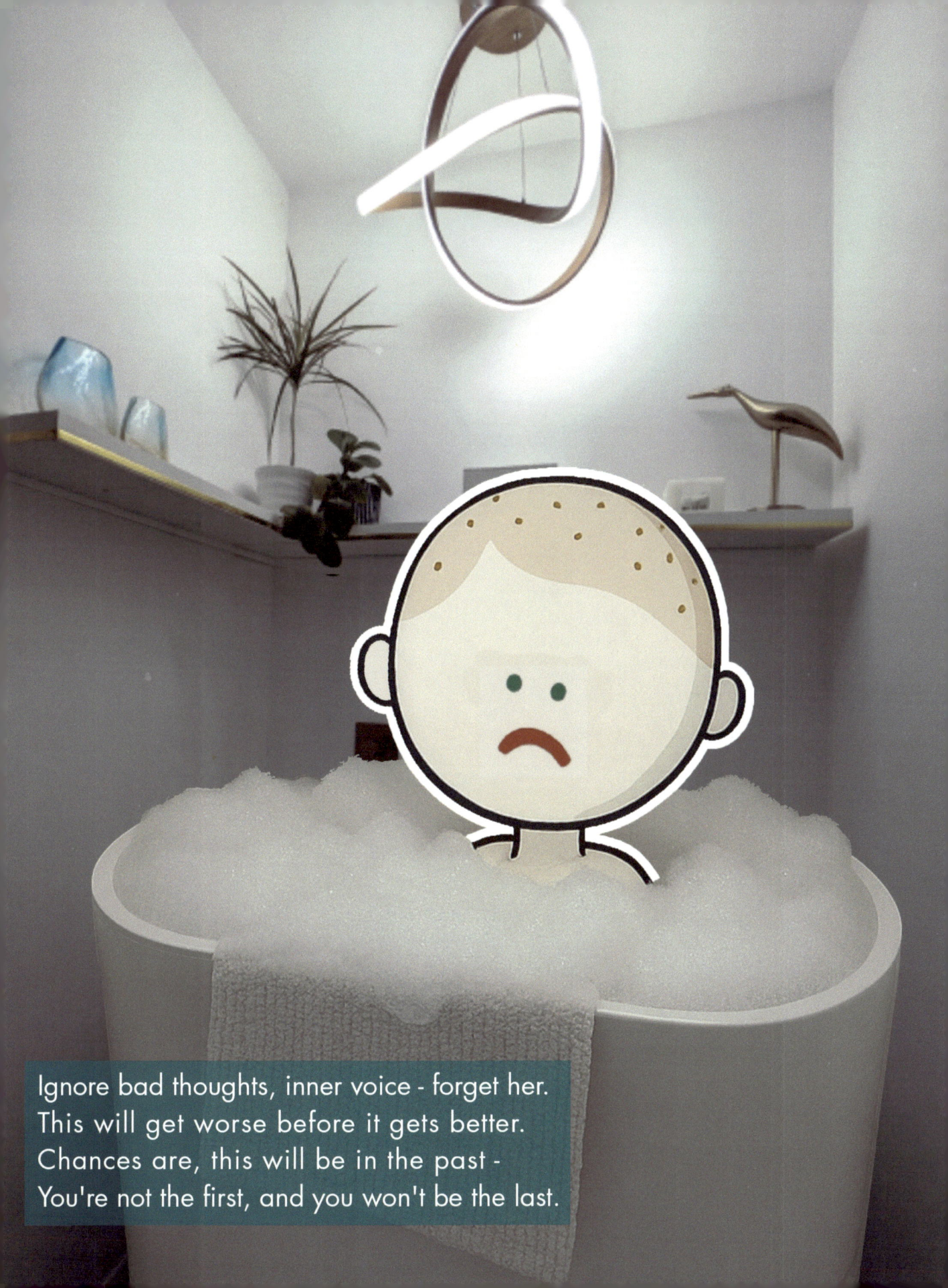

Ignore bad thoughts, inner voice - forget her.
This will get worse before it gets better.
Chances are, this will be in the past -
You're not the first, and you won't be the last.

Things have changed, I'm bald, weak and thin.
But I'm stronger and wiser - this fight I will win!
As I count down the days 'til the end of this shit,
I research new ways to get healthy and fit.

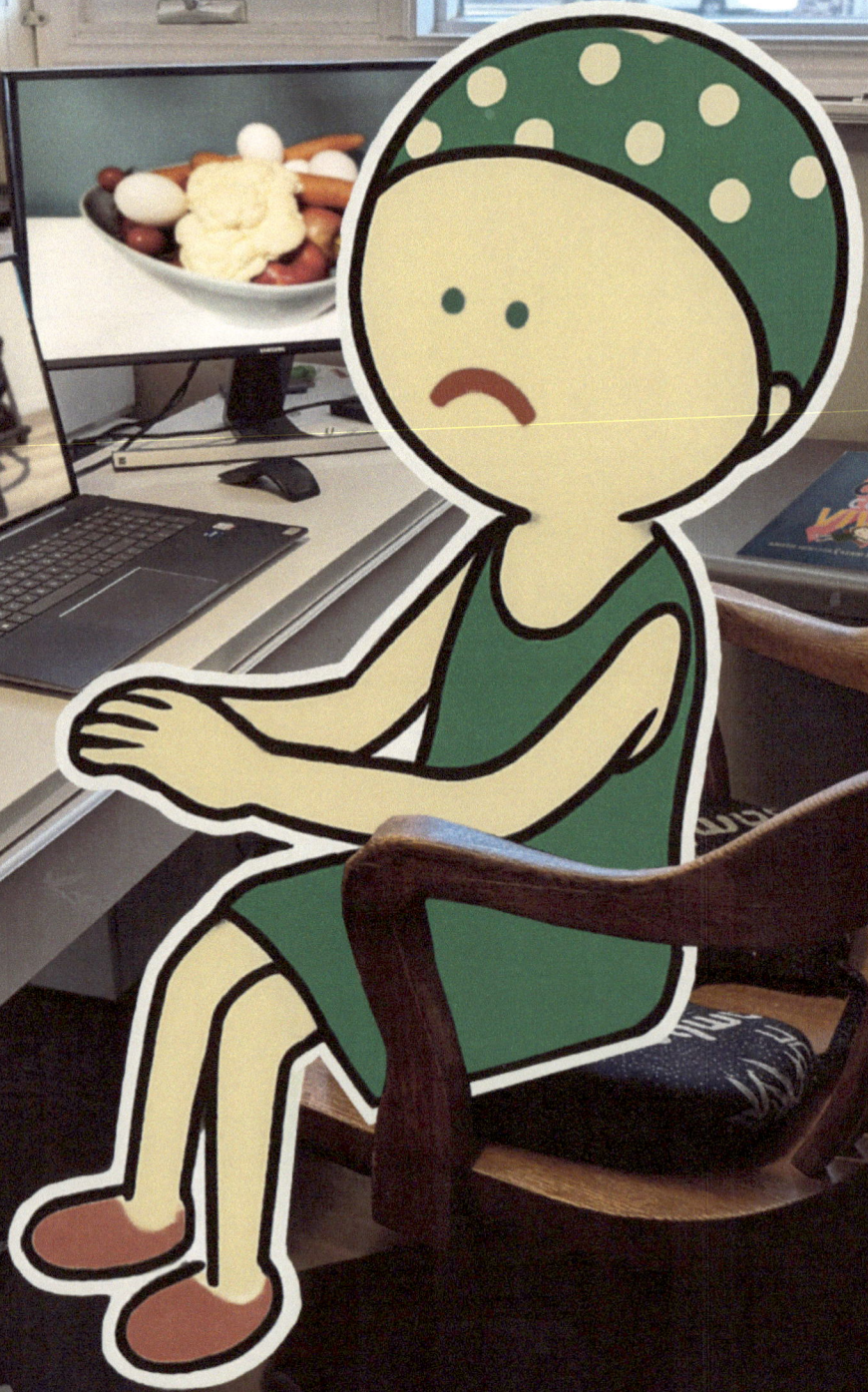

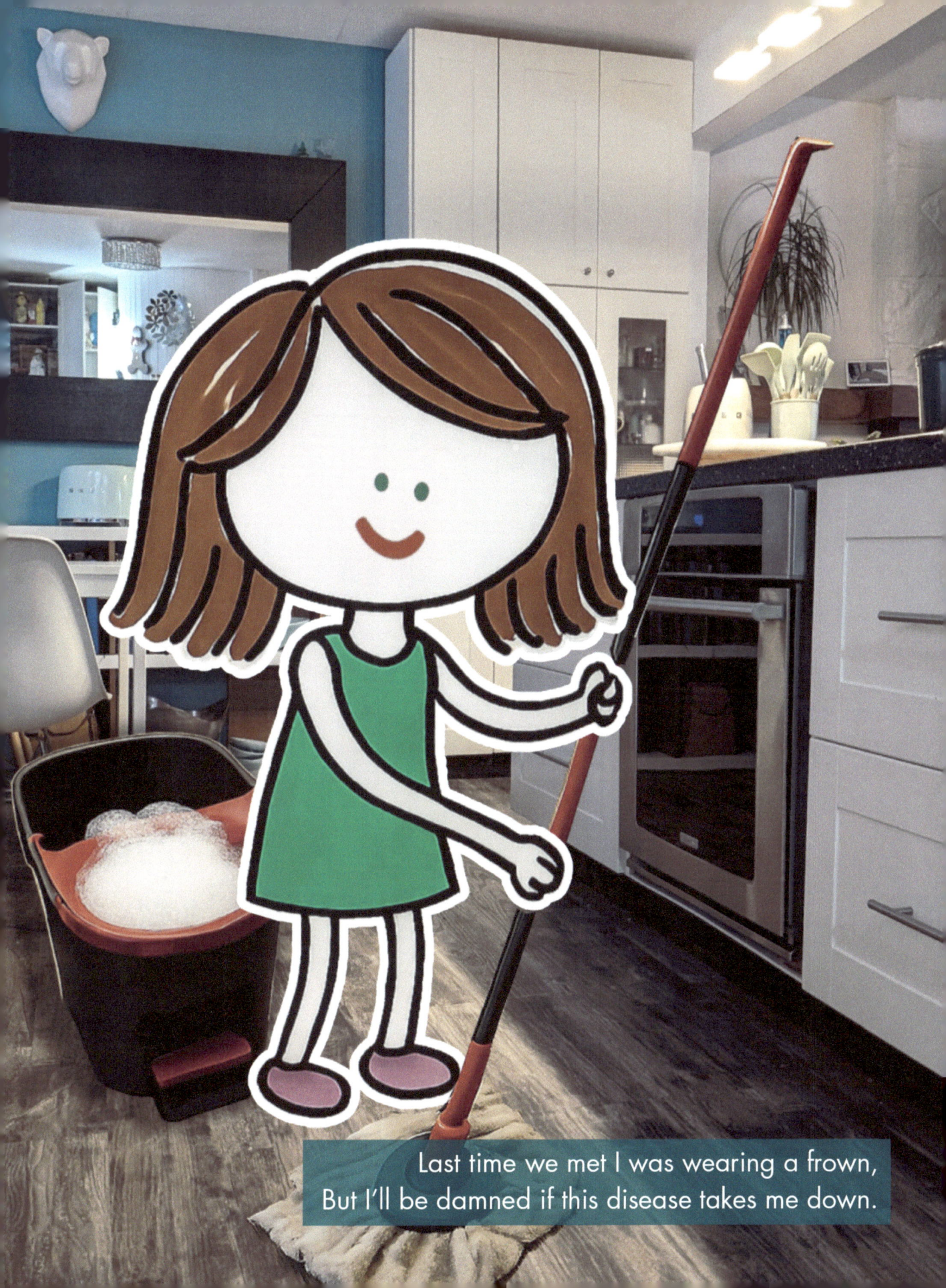

Last time we met I was wearing a frown,
But I'll be damned if this disease takes me down.

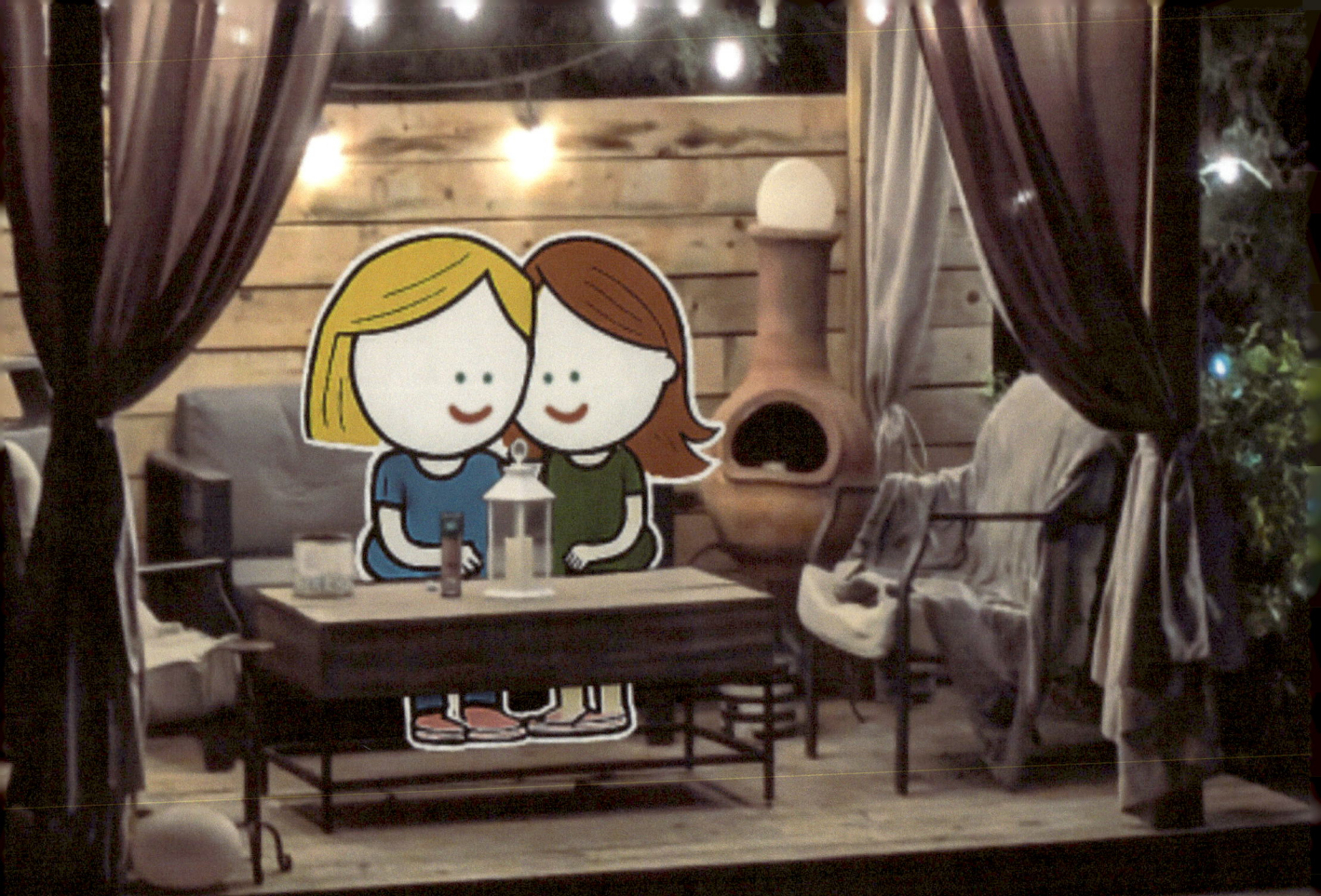

Both my sister and I have been through this shit.
Me in my ass and she in her tit.
Joking about cancer is not the main goal,
But making light of our story - that's just how we roll!

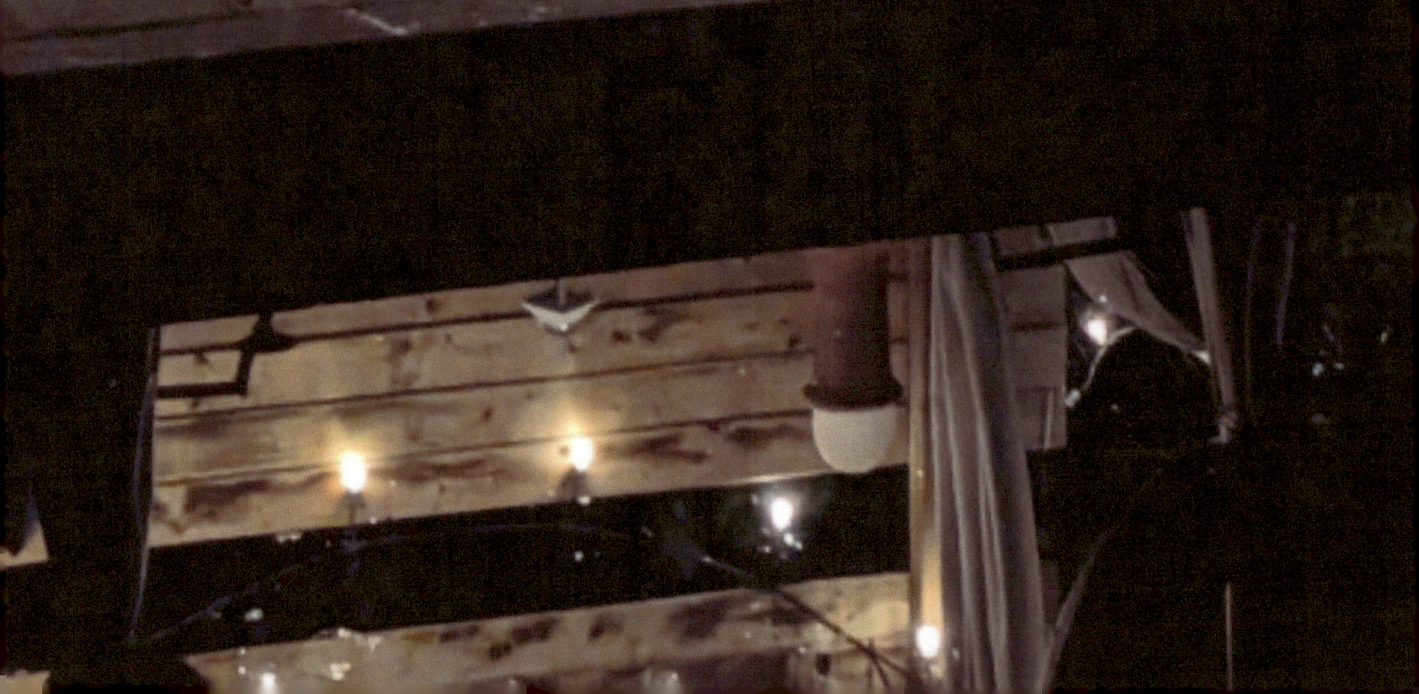

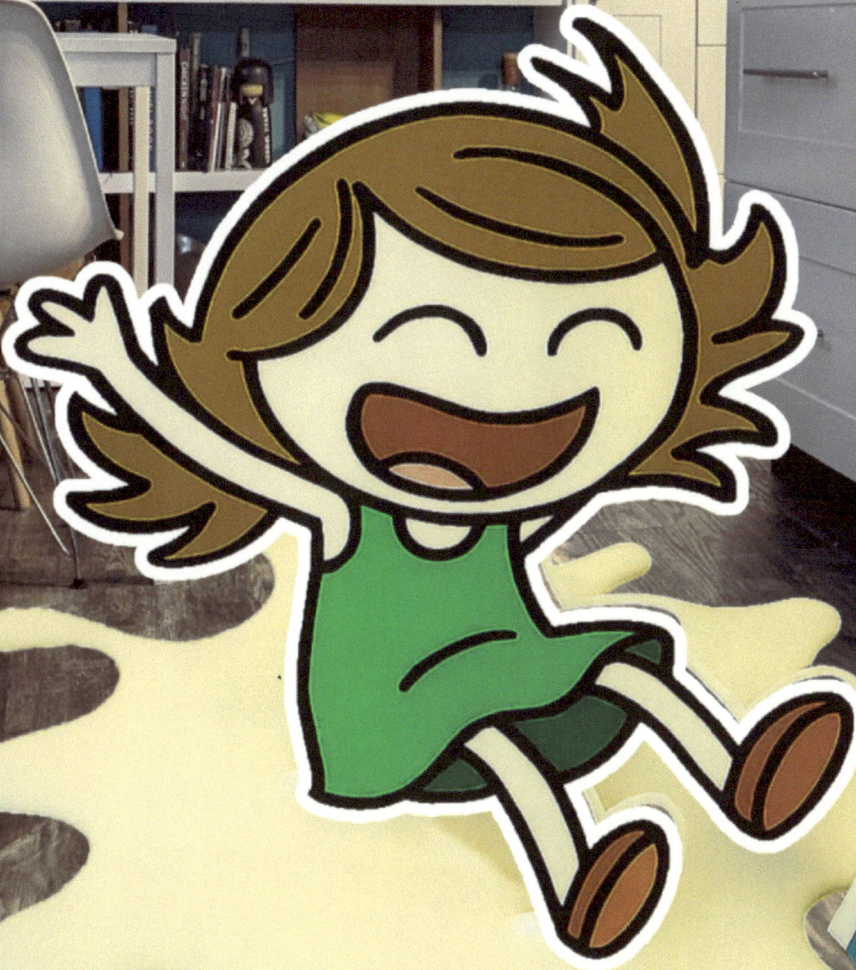

Cancer can go fuck itself in the rear.
Just found out today - I'm in the clear!
All the pain, sorrow, worry and strife -
I've learned more this year than I have my whole life.

Some lessons we learn are filled with despair.
Now you hold life's yardstick to compare.
You'll find yourself grateful for such small things -
This cancer bullshit has given you wings!

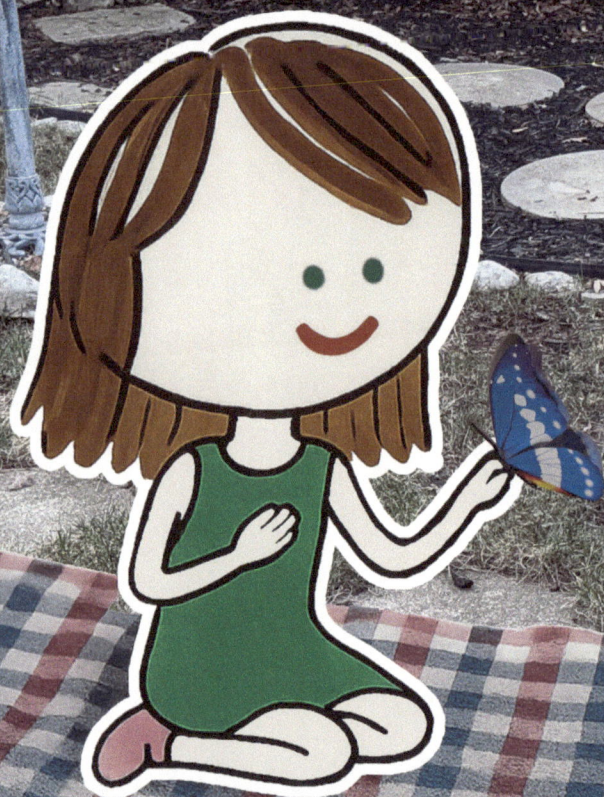

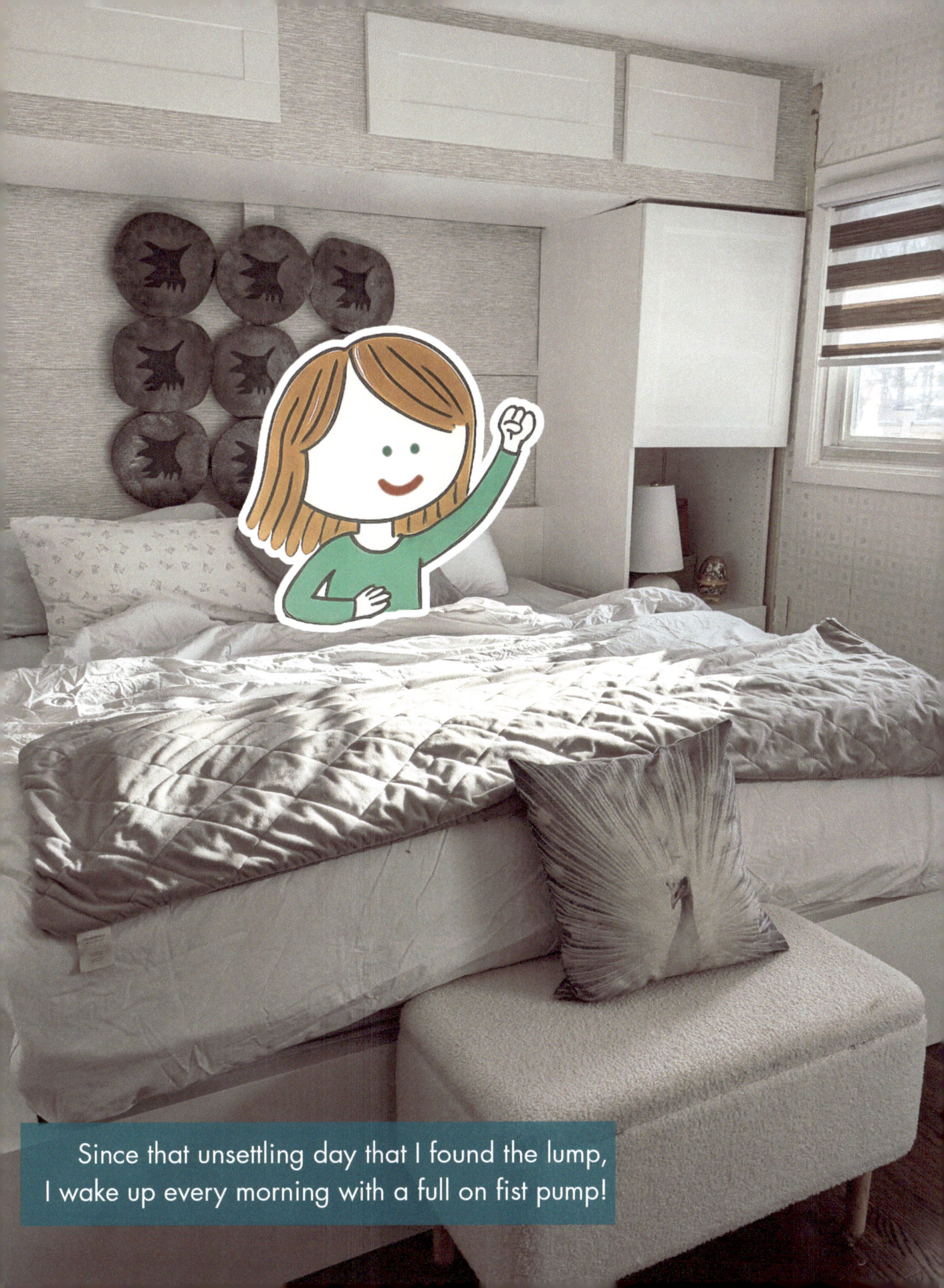

Since that unsettling day that I found the lump,
I wake up every morning with a full on fist pump!

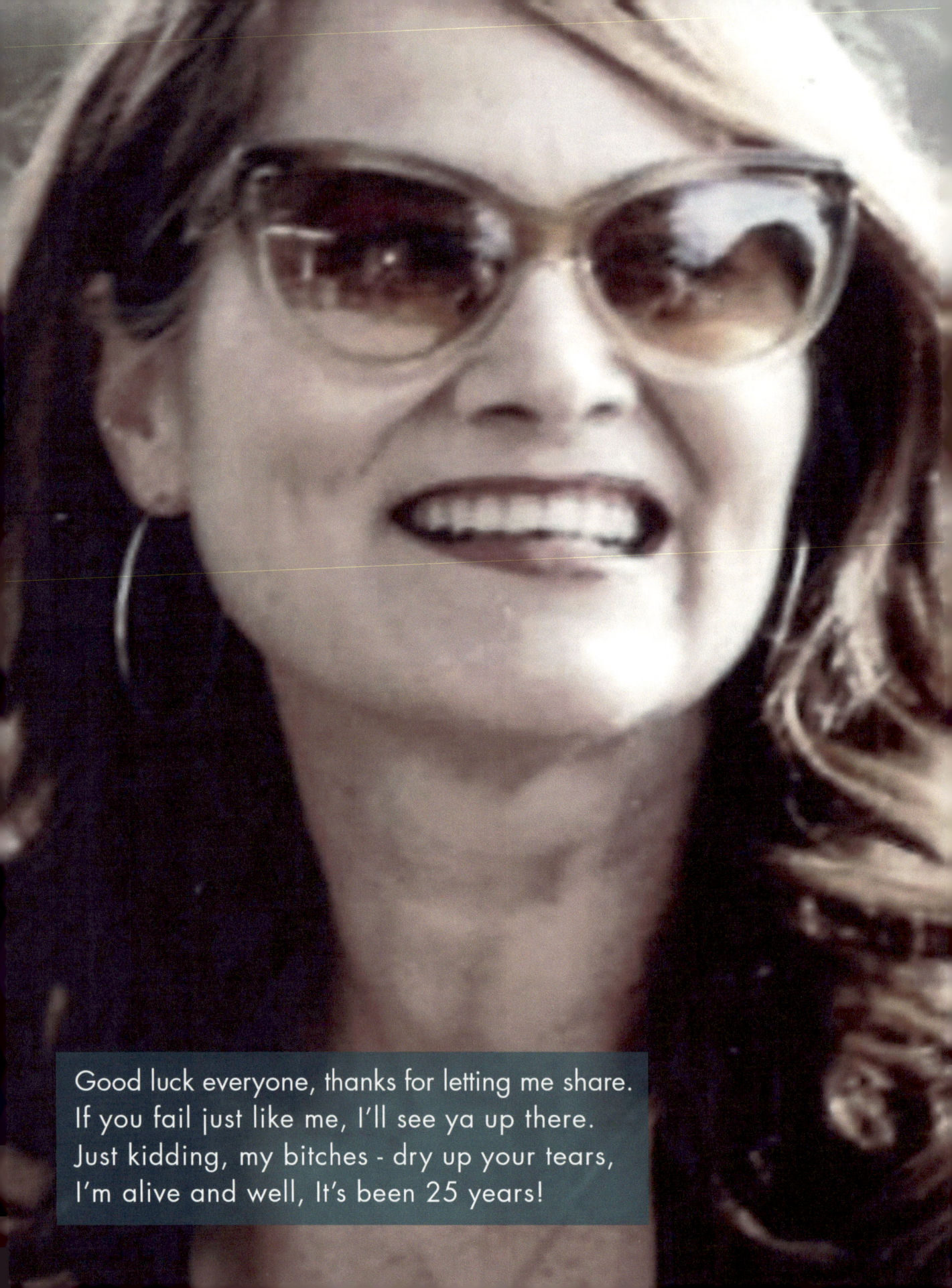

Good luck everyone, thanks for letting me share.
If you fail just like me, I'll see ya up there.
Just kidding, my bitches - dry up your tears,
I'm alive and well, It's been 25 years!

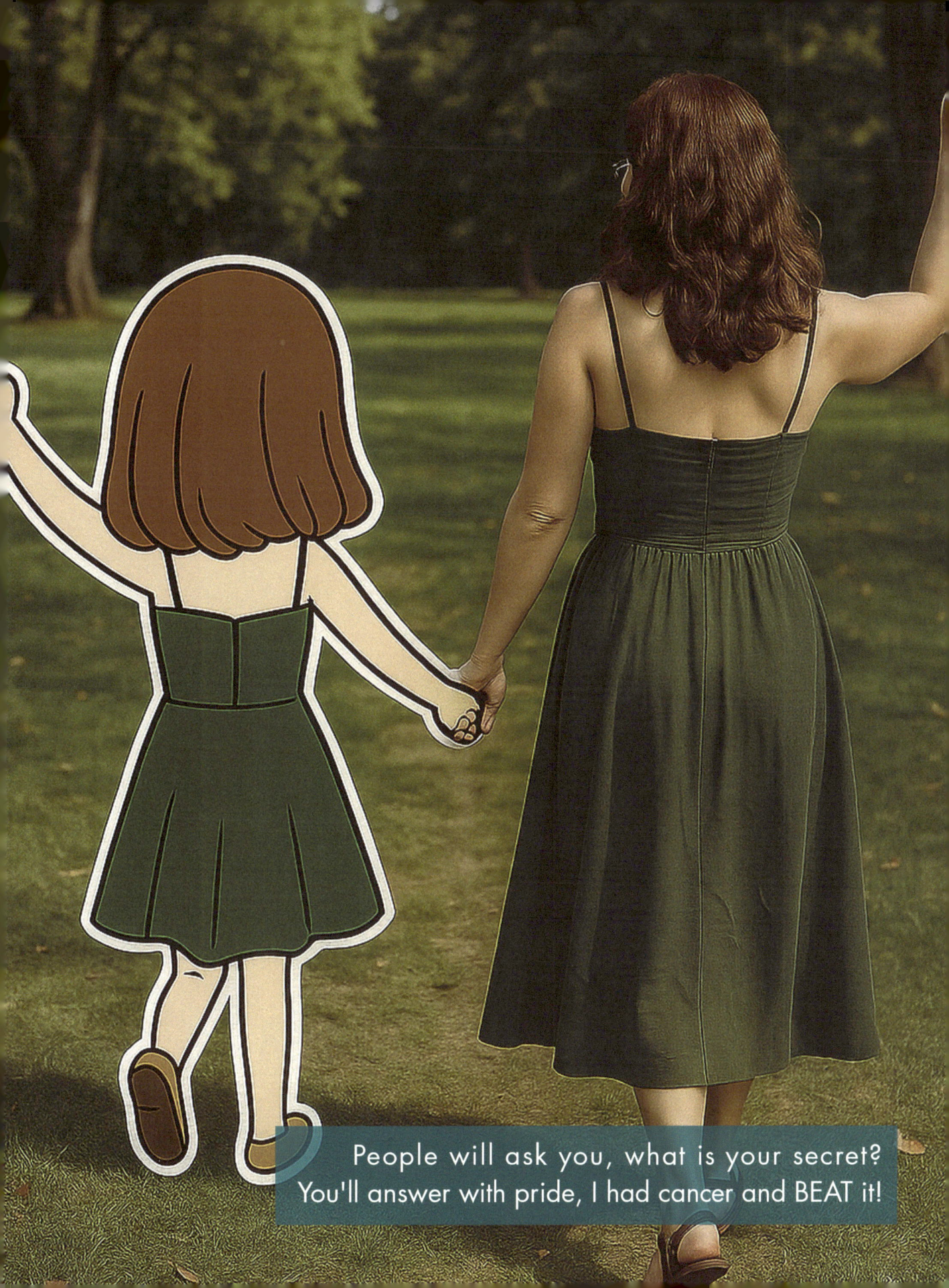

People will ask you, what is your secret?
You'll answer with pride, I had cancer and BEAT it!

NOTES

www.ingramcontent.com/pod-product-compliance
Lightning Source LLC
Chambersburg PA
CBHW041542260326
41914CB00015B/1526